The Stranger Within - (Cancer, the Unwanted Visitor)

~ A guide for cancer patients and their families. ~

Copyright © by Kathy Anne Pippig (Harris)
Third Edition 2014

CONTENTS:

OPENING THE DOOR...

THANK YOU...

The Stranger Within

- Cancer: The Unwanted Visitor -

PREFACE

I have been told and have read in
much of the literature I have
received since April 2002 that
each person's experience with
cancer is different. Each approach
to treatment is different. Each
person's reaction to treatment,
different. Anyone you stand next

to, anywhere, will be different from you, even an identical twin.

I am writing here from my perspective and experiences. I am as different and as *the same* as the next person. We all share some common ground. Certain experiences will be similar. But still, we are unique. Each of us.

What I share here may touch a chord with you. It may speak to you. It may cause you to think you really are different and have you questioning why you're reading this book at all. It doesn't matter. I'm putting it all out on the page to share it. *You are not alone...*

In all the literature I was given to read, I didn't come across one piece, other than a short magazine article, that opened up the doors of a person's mind and heart and laid it out to share with others

Knowing, intrinsically, it wasn't true...I still felt alone.

I'm hoping that in reading this, one person will be touched positively and will be able to grasp something that will empower them, give them strength, and even peace. If I can do that by the sharing of the months with my *unwanted visitor* I will feel honored. Please feel free to let me know... Contact me at: kathy.pippig@yahoo.com

Chapter 1

KNOCK, KNOCK

It was summer of 2001 and I was driving home from having spent a nice weekend camping at the coast. While in the cab of my Toyota truck I experienced a startling pain in my left breast. I drew my right hand to the spot, testing for tenderness to touch. It didn't feel sore as a bruise would. I pulled my shirt away from my body and took a quick glance to discern if there was a bruise and saw nothing. But the pain persisted. I then questioned if I had injured myself while setting up or taking down camp. Maybe I had inadvertently stepped into a pole, the camper's corner and brushed it off at the time. I could recall no such incident, however, and the pain was a mystery.

It radiated from an area thick with masses and cysts. I have a fibrocystic breast condition. Have had it since I first developed breasts. My mother, and her mother, and her mother's sisters also had a fibrocystic condition. My grandmother had had a mastectomy in her mid-life years. Not because she had breast cancer, but because, at the time, doctors felt a mastectomy would be the safest course to take as they felt she stood a fair chance of developing cancer in that one breast. Her sister had breast cancer and eventually died from it. My mother had breast cancer and a mastectomy. She is now a 13 year cancer survivor.

That I could develop breast cancer was a painful possibility I was aware of. However, I did not expect to develop it for another 15 to 20 years. Not at 48 years of age. And I felt, if it happened, it would be the same kind of cancer that my mother had: Estrogen receptive.

The pain in my breast persisted for a few days, then was gone. Having the fibrocystic condition, I am accustomed to running my fingers over a landscape of lumps and masses whenever I do my breast self exam. I am fairly familiar with what is new, what is old, flare-ups and the like. The spot where I had experienced the pain was of a certain lumpy nature. The only change that area had experienced in the past would be to swell, with accompanying pain, then the swelling and pain would diminish.

Having the fibrocystic condition is, at best, frustrating. Breast self exams can be discouraging as there might be changes each month: a new lump, a swollen mass. At times it made me want to never examine myself again because I felt if something foreign did develop I'd never be able to tell the difference.

Each time I did my self exam, I would pay special attention to that area, in the upper, inner, right quadrant of my left breast. For a time, it seemed that the lumpy mass was getting smaller. And where once was a rounded edge, now was a more pointy edge. Then 9-11-01 occurred and I don't recall if I kept up with my self exams, or not. Come the new year I became aware of another change in that area of my breast. The lumpy

mass seemed harder and larger.
Gone was the pointy edge and the
more rounded edge was back. The
area around it was somewhat tender
so I wasn't too concerned. I had
long been told cancerous lumps or
cysts did not hurt. The area
around the lumpy mass also itched
occasionally. I was feeling some
concern, but decided to keep an
eye on it and let it be.

Chapter 2

WHO'S THERE?

By March the lump felt more
noticeable. A bit larger. And
harder to the touch. The lump
moved about freely; it was not
attached to anything, but I felt a
deep concern, and an inexplicable
need to have a doctor look at it.

On 3-11-02, I called the doctor's
office and told them I felt I
needed a mammogram as soon as
possible. It had been a year since

my last mammogram so I was due. My desire to have it done ASAP I could not explain except to say I felt deeply compelled to make the request.

The receptionist scheduled an appointment for me with my doctor for that afternoon. When I got there I explained the situation to him. Told him about the pain the summer before. He recommended that he try to aspirate the lump. He said if the lump could be aspirated I would have little concern. He prepared me and attempted to aspirate the lump. It would not aspirate. He scheduled me for a mammogram.

The mammogram technician asked me the standard questions and I told her my concerns, rehashing the initial pain the summer before, the slow changes over the following months. She made a comment about cancerous lumps not being painful. I explained to her that the lump, itself, was not painful anymore, but that the area around it was tender off and on. She performed the mammogram.

An ultrasound exam had also been scheduled to follow the mammogram. The ultrasound techs had their questions for me. Everyone did their best to sound positive and hopeful. After the ultrasound, they took the results to the doctor on staff who examined the results. The technicians returned after speaking with the doctor. They informed me the lump looked to be a complex cyst. They stated that my doctor may wish to follow up with a biopsy. They tried to reassure me that a complex cyst was not uncommon, but it can present differently than other cysts.

My physician ordered a biopsy and I went back to the hospital where the mammogram and ultrasound had been performed to have the biopsy done on Monday, 4-15-02. The doctor deadened my breast and took

several samples with a type of
punch-gun. He commented that from
what he could tell, the lump
appeared to be a fibroadenoma. He
further stated that fibroadenomas
were benign. That I shouldn't
worry. The results would be back
to my doctor the next day. Two
days maximum.

The week went by and I had heard
nothing from my doctor's office.
On Friday I telephoned his office
in the morning. The receptionist
who answered the phone stated she
would pull my file and get back to
me later that day with the results
of the biopsy.

Chapter 3

CANCER

That afternoon, on my way back to
the office from a home visit with
a client I received a call on my
cell phone. It was my doctor. He
asked me: "Are you in a good place

to hear some bad news?" I pulled over and turned the engine off. The results had come back positive for cancer.

Chapter 4

CANCER WHO!?

My moments before, lucid world, shut down. All doors closed on what had been, in an instant. My world was suddenly a world filled with delirium. What I said, or how I was able to respond at all is mostly a mystery to me. I recall thinking the sun seemed extraordinarily bright. I thought about the people on the street around me, going about their normal and rational activities. And how I felt cut off from their reality. I know I spoke to my doctor while at the same time my silently screaming self was reeling.

I didn't want to be in my body and if I could have run out of, and away from it, I would have. I didn't want to be me because what I had been told was too hideous; a blaring sentence of unfathomable doom.

At some point my conversation with my doctor ended. I then phoned my mother. In hysterics, I told her what the doctor had shared with me. I babbled. I cried. I had lost my hold on sanity. Somewhere along the line my supervisor had been notified of the news. I could have called him or my mother may have, I don't recall and it's not important anymore.

My mother requested that I drive over to her house. I did. In the time it took me to drive from the roadside, where I had pulled over to hear the news from my doctor, and arrive at my mother's I had made plans to tidy up my life. I had decided if I was going to die it would be sooner rather than

later. I would have no one tend
me, taking care of me. I would not
lose my home, my car, my job and
become dependent on others to
nurse me until I died. I would
arrange futures for those in my
care; those I loved. I would
settle out my financial
obligations, write checks for the
final payments on my bills. Make
quick plans for my possessions;
those that might be of value to
family or friends. I would end my
life by my own hand.

I remember when I got to my
mother's she had a piece of mail
for me. A jury duty summons. The
summons stated that if I was
unable to appear I would need a
doctor's statement indicating why
and for how long. I called my
doctor's office and explained
about the jury duty summons. Asked
if the doctor could prepare a
statement for me and that I would
pick it up that day. It was Friday
and I didn't want to wait until
Monday to get the postponement in

the mail. I don't know why it was so important for me to get that out of the way, but it was. Perhaps because it was something of the "real" world, the sane world, I could hook onto to anchor me.

In a blazing, hot rush, I was being assailed by my emotions: disbelief, anger, fear, shock, sadness, helplessness and hopelessness. I rambled while at my mother's home. Somewhere in the midst of my mussitations it was arranged with the doctor that I could pick up the statement from him within the hour. He and my mother talked and both feared letting me drive. But I was adamant that I be allowed to do it on my own. I would pick up the statement from my doctor, then go home.

A quaking jumble of out-of-control emotions, I signed in at reception, paid my co-payment and was told the doctor wanted to see

me; to talk to me before he gave
me the statement regarding the
jury duty.

I waited. I cried inconsolably.
*Surely, dear God, this could not be happening to
me . . .*

Chapter 5

THE ARRIVAL

My doctor, a caring, compassionate
and intuitive physician sat me
down in an examining room and
talked to me at length. His words
were hopeful, positive, honest
and, though I didn't realize it at
the time, healing.

He managed to arrange to have me
be seen by a surgeon. A surgeon he
held in high esteem. It so
happened that she had an opening
on 04-24-02 and she could see me
then. Apparently getting to see
this particular surgeon, so soon,
was a windfall. Somewhere in the

back of my mind something clicked.
Something lucky had just happened
to me. A bit of shiny goodness had
been dropped in my path and I
mentally bent down and picked it
up.

During my office visit the surgeon
explained the options to me. I
could have a lumpectomy, followed
up with radiation. Or, I could
have a mastectomy. The lump was
large enough, and my breast small
enough that to excise the lump
alone would leave my breast
somewhat deformed in appearance. I
had decided before I walked into
her office that I wanted a
mastectomy. I didn't want to have
to worry about the cancer
spreading in the breast, about the
lumpectomy not getting all the
cancer. I wanted my breast gone,
as soon as possible.

While at the office, the surgeon's
assistant checked the calendar and
someone's surgery had been
canceled. I could have my surgery

in that time slot, on 4-30-02. This, too, was an unexpected boon, as the doctor was booked for weeks for surgeries. Another glittering gem of something positive and good had fallen in my path. I gathered it up and stowed it with the other piece of fortune I had collected.

But, it was still there; that unwanted visitor; *cancer*. Like a battering ram, it pushed through my barriers and slammed up against my personal space. And the litany pounded over and over in my head: *Why me? WHY ME?*

I couldn't shut my windows and doors quick enough. At every turn, there it was; my visitor. Occupying my body, and my mind. Leaving no area free of its presence.

A recital of thoughts kept screaming in my head: *This is not fair! I cannot do this. I don't want to go through this! No loving God would treat those he cares about this way. This is unacceptable. I don't have the strength to do what must be done.*

I remember speaking these thoughts out loud to my mother one day. Her response was: "No one wants to go through it. Do you think anyone would ask for this to happen to them?"

Oh, how true! I was so deaf and blinded by my own suffering, I couldn't look at it impartially. It made sense, of course, what she said. But those feelings and thoughts so filled my conscious day-to-day existence, I couldn't embrace the thought that others were going through much the same thing I was. Yet when I took the time to consider that, the fact that others were experiencing similar pain and dark thoughts, something changed. Suddenly it seemed my hearing; my brain, opened up to a new frequency. I began to learn of others, about their experiences with cancer.

Were more people talking about it now than before? Were more people getting it? The unwanted visitor. It appeared that way. I was hearing about it from many directions: overhearing coworkers; some snippet on the evening news; an article in the newspaper or a magazine; friends telling me about one of their friends or family members finding out recently he or she had cancer. *How very sad for all of us.* But I was not alone...

Chapter 6

SEEKING OUT AND ASSEMBLING YOUR WEAPONRY

Lining up your warriors and soldiers. And they may be many. Perhaps more than you feel you can juggle all at once, perhaps not.

To be honest, initially, I had no intention of telling anyone about my worrisome lump. But it became such a heavy and unwieldy burden to carry about by myself I was drowning from its weight. My plan was to go through with the surgery, if I needed it. Take the necessary time off from work to recover then get back to living a normal life. People at work were to know only that I had taken a vacation. At worst had surgery of some sort. Friends and family would be told as little as possible. And, I had no plans, whatsoever, to have chemo, if chemo was suggested. All the more reason why no one needed to know everything.

I didn't want to alarm my family. We had had enough deaths in the family from hideous diseases: cancer, Lou Gherig's Disease, Alzheimers, Congestive Heart Failure, Waldenstrom's Disease. We had lost some loved ones when they were yet young. After they had suffered long years with a disease. We had had our share of heartache. I didn't wish to contribute to it. My mother, most of all, I wanted to protect. She had lost a father to Lou Gherig's Disease, a mother to Alzheimers, a husband to Waldenstrom's Disease. And, she had gone through her own bout with cancer.

But when it came down to it, when I had to open up to someone, it was my mother I called, with regret for the pain I knew it would bring her. I told her I had no one else I could share with. I told her about the lump I had before I knew it was cancerous. And I expected it to end there. It would be something I shared with her, only. But that is not the way it went. She told family and friends. She told the members of her church about my difficulties. She wanted everyone to pray for me. She shared with others what I could not.

After the telling of it was done I went to work to line up my crew: my primary care physician; my surgeon; later, my oncologist; my family and friends, my God and faith; my coworkers and supervisor; support groups; reading material, an extensive offering of literature that will answer your questions and more; boutiques that cater to the cancer patient; counseling, in group or individually; the American Cancer Society; Reach to Recovery, a group of cancer survivors who come out to see cancer patients. They offer suggestions, listen to your concerns, offer you positive and patient support, and they bring more reading materials, as well as in my case, a soft-construction, breast prosthesis for my bra. The lady who came to see me told me of her own experience with breast cancer. *She knew what I was going through.* It comforted me to listen to her and stilled, a bit, the demons playing havoc with my once rational mind.

The lady who came to see me from Reach to Recovery was a beautiful lady with a soft manner, gentle patience, and boundless wisdom.

She gave me her home phone number, her work number, and stated I could call her anytime I had questions or concerns. She talked to me about support groups. Through her I found out about a group meeting designed specifically for chemo patients.

I needed a storeroom and I needed to stock it. I looked to my own inner resources, labeled them and put them on the shelf, within reaching distance. I clutched at all the resources I have already mentioned and placed them carefully in my storeroom. I categorized them and prioritized them and made sure none was hidden behind another. And all those twinkling gobbets of fortune, that shiny coin of yummy delight, that glittering gem of something positive, I laid them out proudly on a shelf set aside just for them. Those gobbets of goodness are reusable. Every time I take one out and hold it in my hand, gaze down at its perfection and beauty I am filled with joy and count myself blessed. I also left room on their shelf for the addition of more glowing treasures--gifts from the Creator. I left the storeroom door open, the light on, turned away and counted myself ready, lucky...blessed.

I will tell you now, amassing your weaponry; your support, can be overwhelming. There were many times I felt I could not accept another piece of literature without shuddering. I did not want to read about my undesirable guest. I did not want to give it power. Power to cow and frighten me. I did not want to face my friends and family and have to speak about it with them. I did not want others to treat me differently: I wanted no pity. I did not wish to see fear in their faces; fears of my possible demise, fear that they, too, might, inadvertently, invite the visitor into their lives just by

being around me. I did not want
them to feel uncomfortable in my
presence...I didn't want to feel
uncomfortable in their presence.

My family had planned a camping
trip to the lake. It is one of my
mother's favorite places to camp.
We go on Mother's Day weekend. She
had been looking forward to it for
months. I did not want my health
problem to interfere with the
camping trip. If I could not go, I
wanted my family to go on ahead.
They didn't.

My mother had also planned her
yearly spring get together. A
party she gave for friends and
family. This party was in May,
Memorial Day weekend, every year.
It is a wonderful party, held in
my folk's backyard. My mother
grows roses. She has hundreds of
them. She is a member of the Rose
Society and has shown her roses
and won ribbons and trophies. My
folk's backyard is gorgeous and
spring really shows it off to

perfection. My mom and stepdad work hard for days preparing the yard, buying the groceries, getting everything just right. The party is an event everyone looks forward to attending. It is a time to celebrate the season and the joys of having good friends and loving families. I begged her to go ahead and plan to have the party. She declined.

I still regret that my family didn't go camping. And I know my folks missed giving the Memorial Day weekend party. Sometimes the support you line up in your arsenal is more remarkable than you could ever have guessed. I know that without something uplifting, without respite, my mother and stepfather felt the weight of my circumstances more heavily. To be there for me, they sacrificed an activity that could have made giving me support easier for them. They surrendered a weekend that would have brought them rest and relaxation. It would have been their first vacation of the season. A time to enjoy the weather and soothe that cabin fever that comes with being house-bound during the winter months.

For what you sacrificed for me, I thank you both. You have been the most wonderful source of support. I know my outlook was brighter because you fought for me, even when I didn't want you to. You held me up with your indomitable strength and allowed me to take the first steps in my recovery. I am blessed to have you both in my life...To call you family, parent, friend.

Chapter 7

THE EXORCISM

Eviction:

Surgery and recovery.

My mother took me to the hospital on that cold and rainy Tuesday. It was dark out in the early morning hours. I signed in and registered. There were a number of tests I had to take and then I was directed into the pre-op room, I disrobed and donned the hospital gown. By my side were my mother, a nurse, and my anesthesiologist. The nurse was like another mother, or grandmother--so kind, fawning over me. Reassuring me. The anesthesiologist talked to me about the procedure and asked the questions he needed to do his job. He then kept up a conversation designed, I think, to keep my mind off things. A nice man. He pointed out another anesthesiologist and told me the man had just finished chemo. He had had lymphoma. He then nodded toward another woman, a young woman, in the bed catty-corner from me. Her family was gathered 'round her. He said she was in the hospital for her first chemo treatment. I began to cry.

Through my tears a hospital worker brought the forms to me to sign. I was to okay a modified, radical mastectomy. For some reason the terminology did not register. I began to panic. It seemed too serious and all-consuming. I was lost in my personal misery. I wanted most sincerely to be given something to knock me nearly unconscious. But I had failed to sign the paperwork and my surgeon would need to explain it to me before I could receive anything to calm me down.

When she did come to my bed and explained, again, the procedure to me, I sighed, feeling silly for having misconstrued the procedure due to the wording on the document, and my nerves.

My mother was all loving, supporting...and so dear to me. A calming word, a soothing touch, a smile of reassurance. She defined, on all levels, the word mother. I wonder now what it must have been like for her. To be there with me for my mastectomy surgery. What was she thinking? Did it bring back memories of her own surgery? I'm sure it must have, but you would never have discerned it from her demeanor.

The anesthesiologist then administered a drug, or drugs, to settle me down. To bring an artificial peace and calm, for which I was very grateful.

I woke up in the recovery room. I don't remember much about my time there. But I do remember people hustling about. Warmed blankets draped over me to keep the chill out. Hearing someone tell someone my room was not yet available. Falling asleep, waking, falling back asleep. Welcoming the oblivion of sleep. Wishing I could slip into the oblivion forever. Knowing I couldn't.

They finally took me to my room. I got the bed by the door. In the bed next to me lay my roommate--by the window. I was later to learn she was roughly my age, someone I had worked with years before, and that she had ovarian cancer. Her circumstances, her hopes for a bright future were dim. The realization was sobering, and though being placed in a room with a woman who might by dying depressed me further, it also reminded me: Things could be worse. A sentence I would repeat to myself innumerable times in the days and months to come.

The poor woman had her own personal demons and they were having a heyday at her expense. It made rooming with her difficult. I didn't get a lot of rest. She was suffering. I grieved for her. I grieved for myself.

I was hooked up to IVs and a machine that dispensed a pain killer at the push of a button. My chest hurt. My neck hurt for reasons I could only guess.

Probably something to do with the surgical procedure. I had leg cuffs bundled around me, pumping air through channels beginning from my feet, then traveling up to my thighs. These were to keep my blood circulating in my lower extremities. Under the leg cuffs I wore tight stockings--again to maintain proper circulation.

I craved liquids! My mouth was so dry I found speech difficult. I was to be given a liquid diet that morning, but the orders were fouled up and I got only a portion of what was on my menu. I developed a debilitating headache and then I became extremely nauseated. The nurse came in and gave me something in my IV to calm my stomach, ease my headache. I believe shortly after that I received some food and drink. Friends and family visited. I was poor company, but I was so happy to see them.

The day quickly passed, the sun set and evening fell quietly outside while inside the hospital lights lit the halls, our room, the nurses' station.

My roommate battled her personal beasts. I couldn't rest. I wanted to be moved to another room, but I knew there were no empty beds. I lay there and I, too, battled my roommate's beasts. When they finally brought me my sleep meds I was grateful. My happiness, however, at the hope of finding an escape through sleep was short lived. The situation in the room was stronger than my meds. My roommate was in mental and physical agony. I asked for more medication, several times. I was given additional meds and I was able to float in and out of consciousness throughout the night.

It could always be worse. It could be me in the bed by the window.

When my surgeon visited me, prior to discharge. She advised me there was no cancer to be found in the lymph nodes they tested. The surgery had gone well and she was pleased with the results. I looked to be in good shape for discharge. She would see me for a follow-up later; call her office to schedule the appointment. My mother phoned family and friends and told them the good news.

I left the hospital and went to my mother's and stepfather's home to stay for about a week or so. I remember feeling better than I had after previous surgeries. This I attributed to the brilliant skill of my surgeon. And to the love, prayers, and support from loved ones.

During my follow up appointment with my surgeon she told me the cancer was not as aggressive as they had first believed. This was good news. They had categorized it a stage two cancer, and she strongly recommended I have chemotherapy. She referred me to an oncologist, and an appointment was set up.

I was mortified. I had not intended to subject myself to chemo. I felt it a barbaric, backward, and *so wrong* a way to treat something. I had always felt people died from the side effects of chemo treatment before they died from whatever cancer they were being treated for. I shared this with her. She stood firm, though, and said she hoped I decided to go through with it--if nothing else, she asked me to see the oncologist and listen to what he had to say.

I did go to see the oncologist and almost a month from the day of my surgery I began my chemo.

Chapter 8

FUMIGATION

My oncologist was a physician at a California Cancer Center, and it was at the Center where I was to have my chemo treatments. I remember dreading my first appointment; my first treatment. My mother drove me to my first session. I walked into the Center, looked around, saw the people in the waiting room--the patients and their families...and fell apart.

I went to the counter to register and couldn't speak. The receptionist gently directed me to a sitting area near the windows. She completed my paperwork there. *If only I could run back outside. Into the sunlight and fresh air, Into the real world--not my world.*

Before treatment I had, what I learned would be routine, to be weighed and get a blood test. I was then seated in a waiting area. The doctor would see me shortly. In a bit I was ushered into an examination room. The assistant took my temperature and blood

pressure, asked me a few
questions.

When the doctor came in I
immediately found him to be a warm
and outgoing physician. He was
friendly, welcoming any and all
questions I had to ask. He allowed
for my tears, my fears, my doubts.
He turned out to be an
extraordinary oncologist; one held
in high regard by the nurses,
assistants, and receptionists who
worked for him. Held in equally
high regard by my surgeon.

Foremost, he was honest. He
informed me that I could walk out
of his office that day, without
ever receiving a treatment and
there was an eighty percent chance
all the cancer had been removed
from my body with the mastectomy.
He added that having the chemo
treatments would up that
percentage. Added insurance, if
you will. I questioned by what
percentage it would up my odds and
he responded: "By five percent." I

was aghast. It seemed such a small difference, but I know had I not okayed the treatments--if cancer was detected later in my body--I'd feel responsible for not giving myself all the chances possible.

He held back no punches. But his delivery was gentle, kind, compassionate...human. And, as if a reflection of his nature, the staff working with him exuded the same qualities. Were it not for the generosity, the goodwill and positive attitudes of my oncologist and his staff at the Center, I would likely have found excuses to miss my treatments. This I know with a surety.

That first day my oncologist guided me to the treatment room. I looked around...so many people! Some did not look well at all, while others did not look as if they had ever received a chemo treatment. What a dichotomy! And everywhere were the machines pumping the chemicals into those people. Folks of every background, social level, age. Up to that moment I had not been overwhelmed by the sense of being in a medical facility. The Center was a beautiful building on the inside, almost luxurious in its appointments. Pleasing to the eye. And pleasing to the body--soft, lovely furniture, thick carpeting. Soothing to the ear, as well, with pleasant music.

I backed out of the room, shaking my head. My oncologist spoke calming words and redirected me to the examining room. I could get my treatment there, in the room, away from the others. A nurse came in with the chemicals that comprised my treatment: Methotrexate, and 5-FU (Fluorouracil). These were given to me in an IV push. I was also to start taking Cytoxan pills for the next two weeks.

I could taste the chemical, or both of them within moments after she started the IV pushes. (Later

I could smell the chemicals in my skin--detect it in my sweat.) Though I had premedicated to ward of nausea, I felt ill and shaky afterward. I was glad I had eaten a meal shortly before I received the treatment. After the first week of taking my Cytoxan pills, I returned to the Center and had my second treatment. I had also gone back to work that week. And so it began...

It was the last time I took my treatments away from the others receiving chemo. I didn't feel it fair to the doctor, his staff, or other patients to use a room another patient could put to better use. I needed, too, to face my demons.

Chapter 9

COPING IN THE MEANTIME

Having been apprised of what chemo could do to a person, the side effects, I felt a little prepared for what might happen to me. I had gone out and bought turbans, scarves and hats, should I lose my hair. I drank copious glasses and bottles of water, as well as ice tea and Gatorade. The liquids flushed the chemicals from my bladder. They also made drawing blood and inserting the IVs for treatment easier. A nice benefit to drinking lots of fluids was that as it plumped up my veins, it also hydrated my flesh. Wrinkles and dry skin became less noticeable. My hands, usually dry and scaly to the touch, became soft, the flesh pliable. I didn't have to use hand creams. Nice!

Before treatment I would try to eat a moderate-sized meal in the afternoon. And drink plenty of water. I had my treatments late in the afternoon, usually after I left the office for the day.

And though I ate the same or less than I had before surgery, I began

to gain weight--another side
effect. Somewhat depressing, that.
I had to buy new pants as I had
outgrown my others.

I suffered from occasional nausea.
I had diarrhea off and on
throughout the months of
treatment. I got a bladder
infection as a result of the
chemo.

I was taken off estrogen pills.
Not because my cancer was due to
Hormone Replacement Therapy, it
wasn't, but they didn't want to
take any chances further down the
road, as my mother's cancer was
estrogen related. So, I get the
occasional hot flash, the
moodiness, yada yada yada. (smile)
I take an antidepressant and that
eases the symptoms some.

I had a treatment on my birthday.

There were some days I was so
tired I considered myself lucky to
be able to drive to work, sit at

my desk and attempt to get
something done. I eventually began
to get Procrit shots and they
helped with the weariness.

Shortly into my treatments I
became sensitive to any food or
drink that was moderately hot. I'd
wait until it cooled down to
partake of it. Carbonated
beverages bothered my throat. And
to top if off, my gums began to
bleed easily while eating or
brushing my teeth, or just for the
hell of it. And I got nosebleeds.

Then I started to get the sores in
my throat, my mouth, my lips. I
was given a liquid medication for
the sores and it helped most of
the time. Though after each
treatment the condition worsened,
until I had to stay home from work
for about three days. Talking and
swallowing caused great pain. It
would have been a good time to
have dentures. At least then I
could have pulled them out so my
teeth wouldn't brush up against

the sores. Needless to mention, I ate very little when the sores were at their worst. Drinking, too, hurt.

About midway through my six months of treatment I developed thrombophlebitis in a varicose vein of my right leg. It was bad enough that after going to my primary physician's office to be seen, I was directed to take myself to the hospital. I did, and spent a few hours there. They took tests, gave me some drugs and an antibiotic. I was released with instructions to keep the leg elevated, take my medication and try to stay off the leg as much as possible for a few days. They also recommended using a hot pad on the worst area on my leg. The heat eased the pain, promoted circulation. It took a while for it to heal. (Four months later, and it still looks lightly bruised.) Due to the phlebitis incident, I had to skip a treatment of 5-FU and

Methotrexate. The oncologist then elected to give me the two weeks of Cytoxan through an IV drip, instead of taking the pills. The side effects that resulted lasted longer and were somewhat stronger than I was used to, but it was very nice not having to take the pills every day for two weeks. Just to get it over with in one fell swoop.

Healing in general took longer than it did before I began treatments, so I had to be careful of injuries. I was also to stay clear of sick people as my immune system was in a weakened condition. The latter was a bit difficult due to the nature of my job. I am a social worker. I see ill people regularly. My supervisor was very accommodating, though, and worked with me, around my treatment and doctors' appointments, and took some of the burden of trying to keep up at work off my shoulders by reducing my caseload.

I was to approach every activity in moderation. Eat well. Drink my fluids. Get sufficient rest. Exercise when I could and was able. Keep the connections to my means of emotional support open and active.

Not long after beginning chemo I became afflicted with what I referred to as chemo head: confusion, difficulty focusing, memory impairment, a kind of muzzy brain thing. It left me feeling dispirited and often witless at the worst times.

It didn't take long for me to begin losing my hair. I cut it short to keep it tidy. I had a lot of hair to begin with so I didn't notice the loss as readily. However, when I was in my car with the windows down and the air whipping through the car, my hair came out as if teased loose by a cyclone, spinning around me. I left thin layers of it around my desk at work; in my bed and on my furniture at home...it just kept coming out, slowly, but surely. I kept cutting it shorter and shorter--just short of shaving myself bald. It helped. I jokingly referred to it as my chemo cut. I also began to wear the hats I'd bought. It was an experience. One that gives me a slight idea of what some men must feel losing their hair. I was lucky, though, mine would grow back eventually. Not so the men's.

But, there was a flip side to this "losing of the hair thing." And that is this: Everywhere there is hair, you will lose hair. A stroke of luck, a shiny coin of yummy delight...I no longer had to shave as often. I didn't have to pluck my eyebrows as often. I, who have always thought my arms overly furry, no longer had such hairy arms. I had also lost that unendearing peach-fuzzy face. Yahoo! I could learn to love that.

Shortly after the mastectomy surgery I purchased a soft camisole at a boutique catering to cancer patients. It was gentle on my skin and the incision site. In the left cup I placed one of those plush inserts to balance me out visually. I wore it often when in public and every work day. At home, or when I was just scrubbing around, I wore nothing, and loved it!

After the doctor removed the drain from my incision site and the incision had healed sufficiently, my surgeon referred me again to the boutique shop for a fitting to get a silicon prosthesis and a special bra to house the prosthesis. The people at the boutique were very helpful and knowledgeable, with upbeat attitudes and a smile for everyone. I felt like I was receiving special treatment every time I entered the boutique--the staff made each visit pleasant and even fun. They have many articles

of clothing for all different
needs and it was entertaining
browsing the shop.

Chapter 10

COINCIDENCE, TIMING, OR DESTINY?

I am inserting this chapter here
because I feel a look at the
positive side of things can make
all the difference on your
perspective of the world around
you. Of the world you must live
in.

I am very much a believer of
"things happen for a reason...they
happen when they are supposed to
happen...this is the natural and
proper order of life".

I will tell of my observations in
a loosely structured list...

I put off going in for a
mammogram, for a number of
reasons; some good, some not. Yet

I wonder if an ultrasound and a biopsy would have been ordered at an earlier stage of the lump's development. I say this because the doctors and technicians all felt my condition was benign: a fluid-filled cyst, a complex cyst, a fibroadenoma...up to the moment my doctor read the biopsy results. Just a thought, but one that sticks with me.

In January I set out to obtain a dog. A dog I had to pay money to the breeder for. All the dogs I had had through the years were rescue dogs, (and I had rescue dogs at the time). I had never intended for it to be otherwise. There are so many dogs out there in need of loving homes no one could ever run out of dogs that needed rescuing. Unexplainable at the time, but there it was. I got a Golden Retriever puppy. She changed my life and I will tell you how in another chapter.

That same January a friendship was rekindled with two people; a married couple, I'd known for years. I had grown up next door to the woman, had befriended her husband in my late teens. They are as close to me as a brother and sister. They, like me, are animal people. It was due to Greg's urging, over a period of 15 years, that I even considered getting a Golden Retriever. They have two Goldens, three rescue dogs, and two rescue cats. Cementing our friendship again came easily, the bonding deep. On the heels of the three of us getting back together, our parents also joined in and we have had several, wonderful evenings together enjoying each other's company over good food and pleasant conversations. It has been great for us all. We have each extended our "familial ties" to include the other.

In early March I received a flyer from the dealership where I bought my Toyota truck three years earlier. They offered to take my truck as a trade-in at high Blue Book. Now mind you, I was a staunch truck person. Felt I'd be one till I grew too old to drive. My vehicle before the three year old truck was another Toyota truck I had for ten years. But for some reason I went to a Toyota dealer and had a look around at the new models of cars, SUVs, vans, and trucks too.

Parked in front of the Sales Floor was a Toyota Matrix. As soon as I set eyes on it I knew I had to have it. It didn't make sense. My truck was still fairly new, in great shape and there was nothing about it I disliked. Plus, I only had two more years until the loan was paid off. After going to another Toyota dealership and some other dealers, not Toyota, I came back to that first dealership and negotiated for the Matrix. In three days I had it. I loved it and didn't miss for one instant my truck. (When I had traded in my first truck I felt as if I had put one of my children up for adoption; like I was losing a limb from my body. A sad time, indeed.) I had also gone from a stick shift to an automatic with the purchase of the new car. It was a breeze to drive, comfortable and fun. As each day passed I loved the new car more and more. And, no, they did not give me high Blue Book (what a laugh), but it didn't matter in the end. I was happy.

In April I was diagnosed with cancer. I was referred to an outstanding surgeon and a wonderful oncologist. Surgery was scheduled fairly shortly after the diagnosis. My recovery was swift and far easier than recovery I had experienced from previous surgeries. My treatment was to take place in a California Cancer Center with great personnel in a facility that hardly reminded me I was there for medical reasons.

My diagnosis came in spring. The weather was beautiful. This, for me, was important because winter usually brings with it a depression I find hard to escape from. A condition many suffer from when robbed of sunlight for long periods of time. With the brighter weather my spirits were naturally higher, more positive.

As soon as my primary care physician found out about my cancer, there was a member of his staff, Tamara, who became like a guardian angel. She called to check on me every now and then. She sent me uplifting articles. She cared and went out of her way to ease my pain and anxiety. I still hear from her once in a while.

In August I got a male Golden Retriever puppy; a playmate for my female; another family member and friend for me.

This list of things fell into place, and to me, they lined up strategically to offer me the best opportunity and potential for a good recovery, on all levels.

Coincidence, timing, destiny, or God's plan?...Maybe all the above. Maybe they are all the same...

Chapter 11

ATTITUDE

My attitude, in the beginning, was one of defiance, anger, and disbelief. I felt vulnerable and helpless. I felt mortal. None of which felt comfortable.

But after a time, the feeding of those negative emotions began to take their toll on me mentally and physically. They were doing me no good. They only served to cripple my functioning. Rob me of any sanity I might yet be able to cull out of my changed life. I wanted peace and serenity back in my life. I wanted to feel and function as normal as I was able. I needed to make some changes in my attitude.

I had a month off from work to recover from the surgery. Though I began the chemo just as I was returning to work, I think, perhaps, this was a good thing. Getting back to work brought a normalcy back into my daily routine; took my mind a bit off the chemo and the situation in general.

Most of my treatments were on Fridays, after work. This was helpful in that it allowed me to get over any nausea before I had to start back to work on Mondays. And while I took Cytoxan for two weeks I also took Compazine with it to ward off nausea. It worked.

Granted, I had to take the good with the bad. I dreaded the days I had IV treatments. As time went

by, it never really got any easier
to face treatment days. But if I
felt up to it, I'd plan a treat
for myself: I'd go to the movies
after treatment. Sometimes I'd
have a nice dinner out with
friends. Or I might go shopping.
Buy a good book and settle down
with it for the weekend.

When the weather was nice, not too
hot, not too cold, I'd take walks.
I love to walk.

That May, I enrolled my female
Golden Retriever in dog training
classes. We went every Monday.
Another activity I enjoyed and
looked forward to. That class went
so well I enrolled my male Golden
Retriever in classes, too. His
classes were on Thursdays. There
were nights I would poop out just
running my dog through the class,
but it took my mind off everything
else. I focussed my attention on
my dog and the instructor's words.
Both dogs took well to training
and I was proud of them. The

classes brought us closer together--provided physical and mental stimulation and socialization for the dogs and myself.

Each year my family goes camping. We have certain spots we love to return to every year. We usually make reservations for two to three trips to the coast, one trip to the hills, and one to two trips to the mountains. With the exception of missing the first camping trip of the year (the one we schedule for Mother's Day at a lake in the nearby hills) I was able to go to all the other places. This improved my attitude immensely. Camping is the cat's meow. My favorite place to camp is Yosemite. We go around the first week of October. Nothing beats camping, for me, except maybe a trip to Disneyland.

Through it all I made certain I did things I liked to do, things I did before I found out about *my visitor*. Those simple activities that made the day a little brighter. I have always liked to make others laugh. Joking around with coworkers, friends, and family makes me a happy person. Joining them in a good belly laugh; the kind that comes from the center of your gut and erupts from your lips with gusto--that's good medicine.

I guess what helped most of all was how I approached each day. Not taking time to visit my unwanted guest; ignoring its presence, I could take it a day at a time. My attitude was healthier. I felt more normal; more myself again. After all, I had excised its corporeal presence from my body. What remained now was a ghost, a bad spirit. The visitor was a mere shadow and a lot easier to deal with. It was losing its power over me slowly as the days went by.

There is a line from the movie: Gone With the Wind. It is this: "Tomorrow is another day." What a fine line. And it goes with my often repeated verse well. Together, they became my mantra. *Tomorrow is another day. Things could be worse.* And I don't mean by that that things will be worse tomorrow. I learned to be thankful for what I had, today. To not worry about the small things and try to tame down worrying about the big stuff. I found that certain things no longer bothered me. It was a purging of sorts. I felt emotionally lighter, freer.

I wrote the following, what completes this chapter, in another book. I am rephrasing it a bit here, but it is essentially the same. I feel the meaning therein can be applied as effectively in this book as in the other book. A lot of me goes into each book I write. A transfusion, if you will. A part of me flows into the words and becomes a reflection of my experiences and lessons learned. The book I originally wrote this for is: *Siren Song*. I won't say more

as I'd not like to ruin it should
you choose to give it a read...

I try not to concern myself with
anything I can have no impact on.
I concentrate on those things I
can impact within myself. And
leave the rest to the Creator.
Life is too fleeting, too short.
The daily things; the chores, the
necessary things that need doing,
the mundane things I feel
compelled to do each day, are just
that...things that fill up my day.

Things happen to us as they are
meant to, my opinion. We can
direct that course down a narrower
road. Keep it from meandering,
taking up gobs of time and using
it up fruitlessly. But,
ultimately, it will play out as it
is supposed to. And it can be more
than just the living of a life. It
can be special, if we make it so.

The tools to transform our
existence into a satisfying
experience are within our grasp.

There are timeless moments. Many
of them. And they blow about just
as the wind blows autumn leaves,
or scatters words in the skirts of
a breeze. The routes of the
pockets of timelessness move by no
planned course. They just are;
like the wind. And they can occur
anytime. Anyplace. They are
offered, and only by accepting
them will we live them. It is so
simple, really. Savor the brush of
high emotion on the face of a dear
one; allow your spirit to be
carried with the wind as it
courses through the trees; open
yourself to all that lives around
you. On that walk you may take in
the morning one of those pockets
may be within your reach. The
window of opportunity to reach out
and grab hold can be as long as
only a single breath. It you
hesitate, you have lost that
opportunity. You cannot say: I'm
too busy now to enjoy that. I'll
wait until the next time. There
will not be a next time, for that

particular moment. Each one if special and unique.

And know this: Each moment you draw breath something divine is happening, and somewhere else, something evil. Other beings are experiencing the most exciting moments of their lives. While on the flip side, other beings are suffering through their darkest hours. You will rarely be able to change or effect any of it. Just know that it is true and when you are experiencing tough times, think that somewhere, someplace, the extraordinary is happening. The sublime. Draw on that. Picture it in your mind's eye. And a peace will suffuse your spirit.

Often the majestic can be found in the simplest expressions of life. In the sunlight cascading off the leaves of a tree. In the meadow, where mule deer nap on a spring afternoon. In the play of a satiny breeze that caresses your skin like a lover. In the cool shadow of an oak tree shared by a squirrel and a cow; both knowing the day is as it should be; accepting that and peacefully relaxing with a full belly--the cow, and a horde of stored food for the winter--the squirrel. In the trees and green grass on rolling hills above many, small hollows filled with autumn leaves and slanting sunlight.

During those times, for instance, when I am with my male Golden Retriever and nothing else matters--I am simply happy to be in his company and sharing the world with him. My joys will seem abounding when my dog and I are doing what seems the simplest things together. During such moments as those, time is not charted by seconds, but by the depths with which I enjoy the experience. When those pockets of timelessness are presented to me, I seize them. Savor them. It is how I transcend the mundane. How I am witness and participant to the

celestial gift of the Creator.
When I'm feeling especially sad,
or happy, and plunge my hands into
his warm fur. Feel the play of his
muscles beneath my palm. Smell his
breath as he pants and our two
breaths mix. I am suffused with
something not unlike an elixir.
Being with him. Expressing my love
for him. And having that returned
is priceless, and I could never
tell you how long such moments
are. Time maintains no constraints
in those moments. Time has been
taken out of the equation.

When I follow these steps. When I
experience such moments...my
attitude has been healed; as has
my spirit. It is what has seen me
through it all, and continues to
keep me whole.

Chapter 12

REST AND RELAXATION
- Plug Into Your Outlets -

Rest and relaxation: I tried to take it whenever I needed it, still do. Though there would be days I felt up to snuff, if I over did it I felt it later and had to play catch-up.

I'd try not to get too discouraged when it took me twice as long to do an activity now than it had before surgery and treatment. Most of the time I was ecstatic I could do anything. I felt pretty good after recuperating from surgery and just about the time I was well healed I began chemo and it went downhill from there. I hadn't felt ill before the diagnosis, either, which made the reality of the diagnosis more difficult to swallow.

If you can't rest physically, you can rest mentally. A technique that works for me--a technique I have employed since childhood--is to blank my mind out. Let thoughts flow freely through it, but don't allow them to dwell any longer than they need to for me to give them acknowledgment before sending them on their way. Doing this is not always easy and it took quite a bit of work initially to master the technique. And, there are days when my mind is in such turmoil this relaxation technique is hard to come by. But it is the most effective method I have to take a mental vacation.

Another practice I find useful is the one of painting mental images--mind pictures. As I would put the words of visions and images to paper, I put them to mind by painting the scene with vivid clarity. Complete with sights, sounds, and smells. I usually visualize the places I love best: the mountains, the hills, the coast, the nearby countryside. A meadow. A lake, or stream. A flower-blanketed field.

On a hot day, the cool, shady embankment of a river. The water filled with colorful fish and pollywogs. The air buzzing with the flutter of insect wings, and echoing the melodies of songbirds. Moist, green grass brushed by the cool water of the stream. Woodland creatures looking on from the shade of old oaks and pines. And wafting around me, the fragrance of the wildflowers that dot the verdant carpet of grass...That kind of thing. I can take those types of *vacations* anywhere; at work, in my living room, while doing yard work, in the waiting room of a doctor's office.

As I said earlier, I love to walk. It is during walking I often use one of the two techniques mentioned above. The combination affords me physical and mental rest and relaxation.

Also, driving my car outside the confines of the city. Driving in the countryside, the hills-- anywhere in nature frees my mind. I get many of my best writing ideas while taking such drives. I keep paper and pen available in my car. When I get an idea I don't want to lose the feeling it evoked, or forget the idea all together. When driving out in nature I can feel the weight of the city, my job, my problems and worries lift from me. It's a feeling that is hard to beat!

Shortly after getting my diagnosis my friends and family urged me to begin writing about it--to do what I am now doing. But it was too raw and too close at the time. The very thought of addressing these issues and realities made me quake. But I did write. Perhaps that old cliché, that goes something like... *When faced with my own death, my life flashed before me and I could see all the things I had wished to do with my life and hadn't...*

Well, it wasn't quite that dramatic, but the impetus was there to do the things that were most important to me. I guess being compelled to admit that I, too, could die, and maybe sooner than I'd like, spurred me on. One of the things I dearly wanted to do was to finish the prequel to my first novel before the year-end. Before that, though, I worked on a second book and got that published. It proved a great form of warm-up and I found myself at the computer most every day adding more and more to the prequel I had half finished nearly two years earlier.

I have just recently completed that prequel and as I write this, it is in the process of publication. Furthermore, I completed it in November. Hoorah!

Writing relaxes and excites me. It is challenging and a wonderful form of escape. Whatever your preferred choice of escape...If it is good for you and helps to make your life a whole and healthy one...Go for it! Take the time to get away; mentally, physically, or both.

Chapter 13

DOWNTIME

Regardless of how well you take care of yourself, you might have the inevitable downtime. It can be discouraging and disheartening...A good time to mentally repeat: *Tomorrow is another day*.

If you're taking chemo, your immune system is down anyway and it's a lot easier to get sick. In addition, you are weaker than you are used to being. And, your emotions might be seesawing, sending you on a roller coaster ride that leaves you reeling and maybe even sick to your stomach.

Whatever routine you have set aside throughout your life for such days, pull it out and put it to good use. For me, I like to get snuggy in bed, or on the couch. Tune in to an old movie on the

television, or read a good book,
Or just plain sleep.

I eat what sounds appealing to me,
and drink lots of fluids. If there
is a medicine the doctor has
prescribed, I use it. If there is
an over-the-counter medicine that
would be applicable and helpful, I
take it. (If I need to see the
doctor, I set up an appointment.)

There are other down days when
music lifts my spirits and helps
to take my mind off my body. And
almost always, a hot shower or
bath is invigorating and relaxing,
at the same time.

If it is one of those down days
where your mental faculties have
shut down and you manage only to
feel slow-witted and brain-dead,
occupy your mind with simple
things. Play solitaire. Work in
the yard. Do household chores. Go
to the movies. Go window shopping.
Work on a project you keep putting
off and have tucked away in the

spare bedroom, garage, or closet. Cook. Write a letter. Surf the internet. Take a walk or a drive. Or, just veg out somewhere, let your mind go totally dead, stare out at nothing, and become a lump...(snicker)...I do that every now and then and find it quite salubrious. Really.

If nothing helps, *Tomorrow is another day!* And as cliché as it sounds, the old adage: *Sleep on it and things will look better in the morning...*sounds corny, but it usually proves out.

For me, and I know for some others, too, *it* rears up, ugly-in-my-face, those days I am assailed by dark thoughts, a deep depression. Images and ideas that come straight from a Twilight Zone, or The Outer Limits episode. I feel enveloped in a casement of deep dread, envisioning negative outlooks for my future, and at the nadir moments--considering suicidal avenues of escape.

Days it seems every where I turn
my mental eye there are shadows,
and in every shadow a monster.
Days I feel I will lose it and the
men in white jackets will have to
come and escort me to the asylum.

Thankfully, these days crop up
rarely. Gratefully, I have learned
my mantra well and do not hesitate
to use it: *Things could be worse*. And
though they seem mighty bad in the
now, *Tomorrow is another day!* And by the
Creator, I hope tomorrow comes
fast.

If I can step back and acknowledge
this dark day for what it is--a
weakness in my overall fairly
healthy armor, I can often shrug
it off as a quirky, pesty day I'll
be glad to have over with. A
prayer to the Creator comes in
handy, too. And I'm not reluctant
to send one up.

Lastly, don't forget your support
system: The folks you have
assembled as part of your support

personnel (typically coworkers, medical personnel, an American Cancer Society volunteer), and your support team (family and friends). If all else fails, do not hesitate to call on someone you consider a part of your support system. At this point you have likely winnowed out those individuals not sincere and of no use to you, and have carefully wrapped up, like a gift, those folks who genuinely care about you and have said: *I am there for you. Call me if you need me.* Cherish those individuals, for you will find no other device, drug, treatment, or escape that will give you what the people who have offered you their hearts, their hands, and their support can. The gift they give you is priceless and the result of your interaction with them long-lasting and deeply rooted in all that is good!

Chapter 14

TIDYING UP AFTERWARDS

I expected that after treatments ended, I would be well on my way to getting back to normal. I figured about a month down the line that I'd feel about like I did before the whole ordeal began.

During a follow-up appointment with my oncologist he informed me it would take six months to a year to get back to normal. I was a bit crestfallen, to say the least. But it made sense, considering all the chemicals they had pumped into my body--all the changes those chemicals had made to my body, my system. And even the effect they made on my mind and, in some part, my outlook.

Nonetheless, there were things I could do to clean up, gather up, and then toss away: the devices and crutches I had come to rely on during my recovery and treatment. Things I no longer needed and perhaps hadn't needed in a while.

The magazines that sold apparel to cancer patients. I could put in storage, or even throw away all those pamphlets, flyers, handouts and whatnot I had been given at the time of my diagnosis. I could pack away the hats, scarves, and turbans I had purchased and worn and didn't wish to wear again (though there were a few I liked enough to continue to wear). Or I could give all the above to someone who would find them useful.

I could stow the anti-nausea medicines I had been taking away, in the darkest corner of my medicine cabinet. Big happy sigh!

The mints, gums, or candies I took while the chemo was being administered, so I wouldn't taste the chemicals. And while they were helpful then, I have grown sick and tired of looking at them, using them, even smelling them now. I can toss those, or give them to the kid next door.

Same thing for the power bars, or
the like, I had on occasion tried
to pass off as my substantial
meal...the ones I may have eaten
prior to getting my treatments. I
bought cases of those things. I
can't stand the sight of them now.

I also purchased cases of bottled
water, Gatorade, mineral water,
and big containers of juices. I
haven't grown tired of them. I
have actually developed a taste
for them. Before I hated water,
had never tried mineral water.
Gatorade I had always kept around
the house and enjoyed. Same thing
for juices. Well, I rather like
drinking a bottle of spring water,
or mineral water on a regular
basis now. Go figure! Oh, yeah,
the mineral water took a little
getting used to. I got the
flavored type, but once I became
accustomed to it, I found the bite
of it refreshing, and, if I have
an upset stomach, the mineral
water settles it down. Nice! And

good for me too. But my experience isn't necessarily going to be like yours.

I could now rearrange my life and pencil in other activities on my calendar on the days I formerly had treatment...the weekends I had set aside for recovery.

I can expect to go to work and not come across those Fridays when I had treatments and found my daily activities overshadowed with the dread that preceded each treatment. As much as I had hated those days, I had stayed the course. I had made it, and I could give thanks that I didn't chicken out and walk away from it like I wanted to do before my first treatment.

I could color my now gray, mercury, and silver colored hair! I felt the gray was growing old, excuse the pun, and I was thrilled to be able to color it again. During treatment, I had stopped coloring it as it was brittle and had that nasty habit of tumbling from my scalp.

Ah, and foods and drink--I can experiment with my old favorites; see if they can be tolerated. Granted, I still have that extra poundage around my middle and the added padding on my thighs, but oh, how wonderful is the idea that I could now, maybe tolerate carbonated beverages, warm to hot foods. And the foods that used to toss my tummy if I took a whiff of them during the months I received treatment now began to smell luscious and inviting once again. What the heck! I'm figuring that it will take six months to a year for my metabolism to get back to normal; for me to pare my weight down to where it was before. So I'm not going to feel too guilty about savoring my renewed delight in foods and beverages. True, I could buckle down, work out regularly...push to get my weight down, now. Eschew the temptations

of food and drink, and eat only
what is best for me, with the
fewest calories. I could...but I
don't want to. Ha!

Before I was diagnosed. From the
time my mother received her
diagnosis I would recoil from the
mention of *cancer*. If I was with my
mother and a commercial came on
discussing breast cancer, I'd look
over at her to register the effect
it might have on her. Time after
time, through the years I did
this. And time and again, my
mother's response was--nothing!
But I was still recoiling just
hearing the word coming from the
television or the radio. Medical
misfortune ran in the family, it
was only a matter of time my
misfortunes came knocking at my
door. And because I felt
chemotherapy was more a form of
pesticide than anything I would
ever call a drug, I cringed when
commercials would come on. When an
elderly woman or man spoke of
their cancer, the chemo they were

receiving and how tired they would get...An ad for Procrit. A death knell for me. I would switch off the sound on the commercial for the Cancer Treatment Centers of America...I didn't want to hear the words--same thing with radio ads. And the commercials about cancer, cancer treatments, cancer drugs, cancer facilities--if felt like they were multiplying like rats--a barrage of them every time you turned around. Was there no where to hide?!

I recently rescued a stray kitten. When I first saw her she looked to be about ten weeks old. She was petite and a little thin. When I took her to the vet he advised me she was about three and a half months old. At home when the dogs would playfully chase after her, she would scurry under my futon bed. The frame is just under three inches above the floor. A week later when pursued by the dogs she would run to the bed and try to squeeze underneath. She was unable to do so and had to face the dogs. She had grown so much she was unable to hide. What happened? Did the dogs maul her? No, they all played together and she has quickly grown to expect play sessions with them.

Well, you know what!? I have faced my demons. I have looked death in the face--my undesirable guest. I have stayed the course with the bogeyman chemo. Now, when those commercials come on, my reaction is--nothing! No need to fear that which I have conquered. I have grown past the need to hide. A couple more sparkling treasures to keep the others company.

Chapter 15

GIVE THANKS

It never hurts to do so, and it improves your attitude, gives you a brighter perspective on your outlook for the future.

I am thankful that...

...God listened to my prayers and the prayers of others, and responded.

...I have friends and family who wanted to offer up prayers for me.

...There were a few acquaintances, coworkers, and even strangers who also spoke some prayers for me.

...I am no uglier now than I was before my ordeal. In that I mean-- I do not consider myself an ugly person. I have, at times, considered myself to be attractive, plain, ordinary, and lovely. Even unappealing at times. I have my share of scars, both on the outside and on the inside. Scars of the body and scars of the heart and soul. But if it was possible to eliminate the scars, so all that remained was a smooth surface, inside and out, I would appear as generic as a Barbie doll. I'd have no depth, no character, no hard experiences to shape my growth throughout life, no characteristics to give me a mature personality, or even an interesting one. I may feel lopsided (grin), but I do not feel ugly.

...I still have my mind, my home, my family, my job, and my loved ones.

...I can still enjoy things like I used to, with a childlike joy and awe.

...Those who care for me have lent me their unconditional support, love, and bolster me up with positive vibes.

...I still have a sense of humor.

...Life goes on and the world still turns.

...My hair is growing back.

...My appetite is on the mend.

...The world around me does not seem ugly, or brutal as a result of my experience.

...I still believe in hope and miracles.

...Though I am less naive than before, I am not jaded and bitter.

...The close friends I have now are the same ones I had *before*. Either they have good judgement, or I do, or both. It is a blessing!

...I feel more mortal than before, but at the same moment, more alive.

*

...I'm thankful I am not in the bed by the window.

Chapter 16

ANIMALS

(If you are not an *animal person*, go ahead and skip this chapter.)

I have no children. Due to problems with my reproductive system I was never able to bear children. At the age of 42 I had a complete hysterectomy. Unless I adopt, I will remain childless. Whether it is a good thing or a bad thing--I will have no children to comfort me in my old age. Not that having a child guarantees that they will love you or be there to comfort you in your old age. Who knows? I may not need comforting in my Golden Years. But it's something people talk about and I wonder if I will regret that I couldn't have a child. Such is life, though. And it has given me more time to spend with my fur kin.

I am an animal person. I have always been an animal person. I shall always be an animal person. I love animals!

Second chance--if you do not care for animals, go to the next chapter. No problema!

I love them all, but I do have my favorites. That being the dog first, and their distant relatives, the wolves. Followed by dolphins, cats, small furry creatures, feathered friends, and even scaled critters.

During my years on this earth I have shared my world and life with most of the animals listed above. Regrettably, but inescapable, I have not spent my days, or even one day with a wolf or a dolphin. Someday I'd love to spend some time in their environment--a dream, and one I shall never let go of.

The furry companions who share my life and world I consider my family, my confidantes, my friends, at times my protectors, and always, they are a part of my spirit and heart.

They are what make my house a home; they are the soul of my abode. I cannot imagine life without them. I personally feel that if a person cannot love an animal, a part of their soul is missing, or perhaps lies dormant.

My companions are what make me more human. In many ways I prefer their company to the company of humans. And many times they can offer me a solace that cannot be found anywhere else.

If I were to lose all my relatives, my skin kin, I would still have my furry companions-my fur kin. My fur kin are what make me whole, they round me out and take me beyond merely being human. They bring me just a little closer to being what they are--something greater than anything human. Something purer and more wholesome, with a boundless reservoir for love and a giving, devoted, and loyal nature.

It is said that being in the presence of an animal improves one's health. Petting a dog or cat lowers a person's blood pressure; has a soothing effect on that person's nervous system. And likewise, the animal can respond in a similar manner to the affections and presence of a human.

Dogs and cats have always been my best friends. They have been an extension of myself. And I would feel honored if, in their world, I were considered an extension of their hearts, and their spirits. When I cross over the Rainbow Bridge, I hope to greet them all, gather them unto me, and become lost in a group hug full of kisses and murmurings of sweat affection.

As I mentioned before in another chapter, the female Golden Retriever I got in January altered my life. Buying her went against all that I have practiced concerning the adoption of animals and bringing them into my household. I had only once before, some twenty-five years earlier, purchased a dog. All the other dogs I have had have been rescue animals. The cats, too. Oh, I've purchased a number of dogs--from the pound. But only that one time did I seek out a breeder. Until this last January...I can't explain why I felt compelled to do it. I *can* say it was meant to be. It happened because it was supposed to. The Creator had a guiding hand in directing my life before I realized I had need of it.

The following paragraph I wrote as a kind of dedication to my female Golden Retriever. You can, of course, substitute any breed name (cat or dog) in the place I have written the words Golden Retriever. *Mutt or Heinz 57* would do nicely there, too.

If there were a Unicorn in the dog world, the Golden Retriever would be that magical being! It may be that the Creator, in his wisdom, did transform that amazing creature's life force, its soul, into a Golden, for safe keeping. For surely, no decent man or woman, would hunt down a Golden. Nor would they imprison one. And in this manner, the Golden did not need to relegate itself to the darkest, and thickest of the forested realms; in obscurity; to be regarded as nothing more than myth, legend, and lore. And as it once was, it is still: only the purest of hearts; those open to the mystical and magical nature of creation are able to discern the cast of the Unicorn. As the Unicorn didst glow; a radiance that shown from within and burst outward round the animal in an aura; a torch in the midnight shadows of the magical realms of yore: So does the Golden glow: For it is sunlight wrapped in fur. And in its presence there is a healing and restoring of the human soul--a lifting of our spirit from the mundane to something higher, more celestial. A Golden's presence is a balm; an elixir. A lifetime filled with laughter; with a playful presence; and love given unconditionally from a heart of purity, loyalty, and innocence. A heart that is finely attuned to the human heart, the human mind, the human spirit: A heart that will give back more than any human could ever repay; so bounteous is the Golden's élan vital. If you have had the privilege to find yourself in the keep of a Golden, you had found your Unicorn.

In this past year the dogs and cats whom I call family have been the sunlight in the shadows of the darkest year of my life. I am very thankful for all of you--my fur kin!

Chapter 17

RESPOND

Respond to your heart, your mind, your questing spirit. Don't let an opportunity slip past you to explore more of the world around you. More of the splendid wonders still waiting to be discovered.

Respond to others who might benefit from your experience. From your pain and your joy. Give them honesty, but do so with compassion.

Respond to your friends and family. They still need you, as you need them. That hasn't changed. It is what friends and family do for each other.

Respond to your needs, be they medical, nutritional, health, physical, mental, emotional, occupational, or financial. Don't neglect them.

Chapter 18

THE HAUNTING
- When spirits go bad! -

In all honesty, while writing this book I have often been compelled to step away from the computer and seek out an activity or distraction more lighthearted and uplifting. In jotting down my experiences I have dredged up misty shreds of the ghost. I've had to peel back scars and peer into old wounds to write much of what I had relegated to the dusty corners of my mind. I had allowed those memories to atrophy and shrivel up and moved on with my life. It's been a bit hard and painful to pull those ebony tidbits out of storage. I had to shake them out and breathe some life into them so that I could look at them from all angles.

That unwanted visitor may haunt you. *It* plagues me, unbidden, at the oddest times. It haunts my spirit, echoes in the flesh of my body. Afraid to voice its name. Afraid that as in the old folklore, if I speak the name of the feared one--I will call it from its dark pool of residence. Even thinking the thing's name might draw it from some murky plane where it dwells in wait. I fear... And that fear opens up avenues of dark thoughts and what ifs.

What if I am not alive next year at this time? What if the cancer has spread? What if I don't find it in time? Who will take care of my loved ones? What if I get so ill I cannot care for myself? *What if? What if? What if?* Dreary and gloomy, indeed! And all of these dark ponderings will get me nowhere. They are of no benefit. Nothing positive came come of them.

I am being haunted by a memory. A memory I have given life and breath to by allowing myself to dwell on the what ifs. When those thoughts assail me, that is the

time to redirect my thoughts. Or
just shut down for a while--like
C3PO, the robot in the Star Wars
movies.

I liken it to watching a movie
that leaves me shaken, wrung out
and unable to utter a coherent
word. It is usually at such times
that I wonder if the cure might
not be a good Disney movie. One of
the animated ones, or a comedy.
They are usually quite good at
picking my spirits up.

Likewise, when haunted by *it*, I
redirect my thoughts and energies
to the wondrous, positive, fun,
and uplifting. I look to laugh,
relax, and feel at peace. I look
to envision the world inside me in
an optimistic light. Being
positive can hurt nothing, and the
benefits are unlimited.

I remember and recite my mantra. I
gather unto me those things that
make my life feel special: my
family--both skin kin and fur kin;

my friends; my hobbies. I take
time to do the things that I
enjoy. I don't worry about the
little things--the in-the-end
insignificant worries and
concerns.

I love to write, read, listen to
music, watch certain cable
channels, spend time with family
and friends, go camping, go
fishing, take a walk, go for a
drive, spend quality time with my
at-home companions, crochet, take
in a movie--preferably a matinee,
play my musical instruments, sing-
-to myself, dance in my living
room, window shop, work in the
yard, create graphics on my
computer, email friends and family
out-of-town, surf the internet,
and on.

I like to look at the things I
have done. I used to paint:
watercolor, oils, and acrylics. I
did some woodcarving. I finished
several ceramic projects. I've
drawn most of my life: pencil, and

colored pencils--I still occasionally do some drawing. I used to do needle work. As I said, I like to look at those things I have done. Actually doing them made me a nervous wreck! I was too picky and meticulous. My shoulder muscles would bunch up and ache. My patience would wane. My creativity would shrivel up when I pushed myself to finish a project. Now, I look and enjoy. I'm no fool. I'll stick to the things that are satisfying and rewarding, and, leave me smiling instead of grimacing.

What is special to me may not be special to you. But you know what pleases you. What gives you personal satisfaction. Then again, there may be something you have dreamed of doing and put off. Now might be a good time to look into that dream. I have a few of my own that yet beckon to me: skydiving, scuba diving, taking a ride in a hot air balloon, traveling out of

country, visiting friends in
Australia.

I recall my primary care physician
saying I should look at my
circumstance--having cancer, as
positively as I could. That it
might present me the opportunity
to see the world around me in a
new light. With a greater
appreciation for life. At the time
if felt so cliché and I remember
wanting to scream at him... *My life is
falling apart and you are telling me to smell the
roses!?*

When I think back on it now and
analyze it objectively, I'd have
to say I've done pretty well in
the appreciation department.
Losing a handful of loved ones
early on in life made me face the
frailties of the human body and
the strengths of the human spirit.
I learned early to cherish the
remarkable and the common. To not
take life and its blessings
lightly. To find the beauty in the

seemingly insignificant moments.
So I had a leg up, as it were.

But in another sense, his words
brought home something else to me.
That in my appreciation of life, I
had learned to allot more time to
the appreciating of it, and a lot
less time to the moments of
negativity. This shifting of my
energies has lifted me up on many
a down day. It has lightened my
load and given me more time to
spend living life with a smile.
And ever since that day in his
office, his words have echoed
repeatedly in my mind. What he
said was prophetic, just maybe in
a sense other than what he had
hoped to convey to me. So...he was
right!

***

When haunted, I have a routine I
use that works for me. It is
another one of those exercise
things. If it works for you,
great! If not (shrug) you'll find

something that works for you, if you want to bad enough...

The elaborate version: I slow and calm my breathing and picture a beautiful, grassy meadow, with a bubbling creek winding through golden aspens and fragrant eucalyptus trees. Monarch butterflies fill the air and colorful birds decorate the trees as they spill out their trilling songs. The sky over the meadow is a clear cornflower blue and vibrantly colored flowers carpet the grass below. The smells of the warming earth, vegetation, and fragrant blooms impart a spicy and heady fragrance to the glen. Encircling the meadow is a high stone wall with only one door, of heavy iron.

I am outside the wall, trembling and cold, several yards away from the entrance. I cast a glance behind me and espy the dark, roiling spherical miasma (which represents the embodiment of my

undesired thought, fear, or
horror) racing toward me. The land
outside the sheltering wall is
gray and gloomy. Fog blankets the
ground and the sky is like a sheet
of steel bearing down on me.
Without sparing the time for a
second glance behind me, I sprint
to the iron door, jerk it open and
run inside. As I turn to slam the
heavy door closed, I see that the
ugly, boiling orb is nearing the
threshold, only seconds away.
Throwing my body's weight at the
door, I shut it and quickly throw
the restraining bar across it. At
that instant the iron door
resounds with a deep clanging thud
as the sphere throws itself
against the other side.

There is a small peephole in the
door and I watch as the sphere
batters the door repeatedly,
losing force and substance with
each attempt at entry into the
impenetrable, fortressed wall.

Turning away from the door, I walk out into the glen. As the thudding dies away, the peace and beauty of the meadow envelopes me. A golden warmth suffuses me from limb to limb, and flows through my body like liquid.

The short version: I am in my bedroom (don't ask me why the bedroom, instead of the living room or the kitchen--I can't answer that one), it is night and coming toward me from a darkened corner is the embodiment of my dark thoughts. As it nears me, I reach out and quickly grab the roiling, spherical miasma and hold it out from my body in one tightly grasped hand. I open the bedroom window with the other hand, and swiftly toss the sphere out the window. I slam the window shut and lock it, too. Through a slit in the curtains I can see the black ball pounding at my window. I turn away, listening to the diminishing thuds...then the silence. My window can be opened only by me. I am safe. The dark creation of my thoughts dies in the night.

Chapter 19

OPENING THE DOOR...

...And opening your eyes, and looking out. Boy, those first glimpses of the outside world can give you a fright. Suddenly, you are back in the real world...the one you left when the doctor told you you had cancer.

Does it look different? It's not, but you are. A bit stronger. A bit wiser. You know yourself better now than before. You are becoming your own best friend. Hopefully, you are proud of what you see of your world, your inside world. It will make the transition to the outside world so much easier.

When I returned to work I wasn't certain what to expect. Would I be able to function as I had before?

I knew once the chemo started I wouldn't be up to my usual par. What I questioned was whether I could make it through the day and still come out of it feeling like my old self. Would I walk into the office a stranger? All these silly thoughts circled 'round in my head. I decided my wondering about it was making me feel crazy. So...I reoriented my thinking. How obvious! I couldn't be anything else *but* myself.

It was good to be back at work. To get back into the routine. It was normal. I began to feel quite my regular self, like I had before I was diagnosed. When I got home I had my usual chores to do, errands to run, then I could relax for the rest of the evening.

After the six months of chemo treatment ended my friends and family would comment: "I'll bet it feels great not to have to go to any more treatments!" "At least you are through with *that*." "The worst is behind you!"

Yes, I had said the same things to myself. But the memories of chemo I had also assigned to an obscure cranny in my mind--banished them. Left them to rot and dwindle with the other darkling experiences and memories. After a while it seemed almost trivial to even discuss the subject--I was going on with my life. I was leaving that behind me, making room for brighter experiences and new memories.

Once out the door, I take more time to see everything good and wondrous. In doing this I am more relaxed, more at peace. I linger longer doing the things that make me happy. I try now to look even more diligently at the *big picture* and my place in it. In some ways it makes me feel smaller. But that's okay. My world takes on a more realistic bent, with straightforward expectations for myself. The weight upon my shoulders is lighter now than before. And my *failure rate* is much smaller.

I find more peace in the quiet moments now than I used to. I don't have to fill up what used to feel like voids. And those moments are much diminished, when twilight broke into night and panicky feelings would bud in the silent moments I had to myself.

I'm not so quick to anger: to honk my horn at a discourteous driver, to bristle up when someone says an unkind word or two to me, to fire off my mouth when things get ugly at work, to mumble my dissatisfaction at the action of a family member... Not that I was Ebenezer Scrooge before all this, I wasn't. But I had a quicker boiling point than I do now. I've always had a temper, but have worked on it through the years; taming it, reshaping it. It takes a much hotter fire now to spark it off. Conversely, I don't require that an experience, a moment, an interaction with another, blind me with its brilliance before I take a moment to appreciate it. Nor does that experience or moment have to be as large as before. Wonder and joy come ofttimes from the smallest things.

Chapter 20

STEPPING OUT

Your outset: It is a new beginning. Take advantage of it. I bought new makeup, colored my still short and thin hair, rearranged the furniture in the house, bought some things I have always wanted and never got-- nothing necessarily expensive. At least I didn't go into debt purchasing these things. I have rearranged my life to allow more time to write. I have a digital camera and I am still like-a-kid-happy taking pictures with it, pleased with the results.

Your outlook: Mine has changed. My world has brightened noticeably. How I view my friends and family has changed and I am satisfied to find myself in their company, no matter what we are doing together. I feel freer to joke, freer to voice my mind, more comfortable in their presence now than before and in a way that is easier and healthy. I still look forward to the holidays, the camping trips, the family get togethers, spring and autumn--my favorite seasons, a good rain storm, going to play in the snow in the mountains, bike riding along the American River with my brother who lives in Davis, taking walks with my mother, coming home everyday to my fur kin, stepping back after I've washed my new car and going-- ahhh!, homemade ice-cream, popcorn, a new movie release, a good book, those days I can glance east and see the Sierras on a clear day (rare around here), a night sky full of stars and the

Milky Way Galaxy, meteor showers, and comets, and eclipses. I like that I'm getting stronger. Carrying my load at work is getting easier and easier. I consider myself blessed that I have friends and family who genuinely love me and care about me and want to be there for me.

Your outcome: Instead of taking my life in chunks of days or months, I now take it a day at a time. I find I can fill more into each day doing it that way. If I'm not worrying about the future as much, I can use that energy and time to enjoy the present. Do I still worry about my future? You bet. But I realize I have no impact on the things I cannot change. Little impact on the things I might or might not be able to change on the morrow. I can best serve myself by focusing on my moment to moment existence. I hope I can stay the course: Stay strong. Be happy with myself and who I am. Find fulfillment in the little

experiences as well as those of
great magnitude.

Outlast: I hope to outlast my
fears and worries. I hope to
outlast my expectations, putting
no limits on myself, on what I do
and what I can do. I want to stay
ahead of my ghosts, eventually
putting enough distance between
them and myself, that they are
lost to the past. I wish to
outlast the current methods of
cancer treatment. I want to hear
the word chemotherapy as a term
used to describe treatment methods
of yesteryear. I'd love to hear
about a new, near-miraculous
treatment for cancer that does not
poison a person's body. I'd love
to outlast cancer: To advance to
the day where cancer is listed
among the diseases for which cures
have been found.

Your outreach: So much was given
to me this past year. Folks who
extended themselves for me. They
gave me hope, strength, support,

assistance. They prayed for me and sent positive vibes my way. People from work, from the Treatment Center, from my doctors' offices, from the Cancer Society, from the boutique where I shopped for my apparel and prosthetics, from my family, from my friends, from my neighbors, from strangers in the church my folks attend, from people in the dog training classes, from the dog trainer, from the internet. They have fair filled me up with good and positive things. I'm bursting with the gifts they bestowed on me.

One thing that has always tickled me is to give presents to other people. I get more a kick out of watching them open their gifts then I do from receiving gifts. At Christmas I'd rather sit back and watch everyone else open their gifts. It fills me with a deep satisfaction. Oh, I like opening my own gifts, but I get more of a thrill watching them, especially if the gift they are opening is from me. Likewise, I want to give back to others some of what they have given me. And I want to reach out to others who are in the situation I have been in and extend myself--give them a reason to hope, pray for them, send them positive vibes, offer them a bit of myself--in the form of this book--and pray that in reading it they are lifted up. In reading it they begin to feel empowered and hopeful. In reading it they gain strength from within to battle their own fears and demons. I want them to notice the glistering object that lies in their path. I want them to bend down and clutch each sparkling gobbet of goodness and store it someplace they can access easily. I want them to know: *They are not alone!*

Your outlets: I have amassed a few, and discarded some old ones that I could no longer plug into (the power source to them had been cut off). My outlets are vital to my existence. My living a happy, wholesome, fulfilled life. I have mentioned most of them already. My outlets are spiritual, physical, mental, emotional, some even tangible.

Spiritual: Not everyone prays to the same god. Some do not pray to a god at all. I do. Raised Christian I attended church growing up, and, as a young adult. As an adult I draw upon much of what I learned in the church and in various Christian youth groups I participated in. I have studied other religions and there is much in each belief structure that is good and can teach a person many things to help them live their life. I cannot say that I subscribe to any religious denomination, per se. I do not condemn other people's beliefs. Nor do I preach my beliefs. I choose to live my life according to the belief structure that works for me. I broaden my definition of God to encompass the earth and all upon it. The Creator, to me, is in all things. I champion causes that work for the betterment of our environment and the creatures we share our world with. I pray to the God in heaven, and I respect God's creation that is my world. The planet I have the privilege to share with wondrous creatures and landscapes of countries and continents that are beyond description in their beauty.

Physical: I have enjoyed certain physical activities through my life. I love horseback riding, had a Quarter Horse mare at one time and I was in heaven. I love to swim, but the water can't be cold. I'm weird like that. Cold water hurts my body. But I can swim till my skin shrivels up and I am chlorine-blind. A warm lake is paradise. A cool river, too, if the temperature outside is crisping my skin, nothing beats the feeling of jumping into a cool, burbling river. Walking. I have always loved to walk and I hope that never changes. I *hate* to

run. But fast-paced walking is a
breeze. A slow, leisurely walk is
oh-so-nice. I enjoy doing yard
work. I like being out there in
the dirt, the grass, among the
trees and shrubs and plants. I
like how the yard looks after I
have worked in it. That I like
yard work is not a statement I
would have made about eight years
ago. I hated it. When I purchased
my house, I had them build the
model I selected on a larger lot
for the sole purpose of giving my
dogs room to run and play. Not for
the purpose of keeping up a yard,
for the planting of trees,
flowers, and shrubs. But something
happened. I became obsessed rather
quickly. In no time I was eagerly
driving to nurseries; to Home
Depot, to Orchard Supply, and to
Walmart to shop in their
nurseries. I began to read up on
plants, trees, shrubs and flowers.
I selectively chose what I planted
in my front and back yard with
glee. I discovered the joy of
statuary and found pieces that

were just right for the yard. I did all this until I had no spare piece of dirt left. I had even dug up portions of my yard so I could plant something. Scary! I look forward to hiking when we camp in the mountains, the hills, or the coast. Oh, not the kind of hiking that requires backpacks and hiking boots and a plethora of finely toned muscles and a never-ending supply of hutzpah. And certainly no hiking that would take me to a place of dizzying heights above perilous drops where the people below are specks. Bike riding is often fun and it is good exercise. I long ago gave up the bikes with multiple gears and squeezable brakes. I have an old fashioned cruise bike. The kind you stop by pushing the pedals backward with your feet, and the only gear available is the "torture when climbing uphill" gear. I get off and walk the bike if the ascent is too steep. But I feel like a kid when bike riding. Badminton is physically demanding, rather like

aerobics. I have played badminton
since I was a little kid. I
usually play with my brother, and
family, when we are all together.
We have our own rules, family
rules. We can be relentless.
Fishing. I don't get to do it that
often. It is an activity I learned
at my father's side. He'd take my
brother and me fishing on a
regular basis. He taught us
everything we know. I still have
mental pictures of the three of us
at the lake, or the river. They
are memories suitable for an oil
canvas, paints, and brush. We
spent many a warm, summer evening
trekking the shore of the local
lake, or threading our way through
reeds and water plants edging the
river in the hills south of town.
The lap of waves against the lake
shore. The buzz of dragonflies in
the air. The scurry of animals in
the bushes and outcroppings of
rock. The smell of water, moist
earth, and sun-warmed vegetation.
The splash of a fish cresting the
surface of the lake. The

camaraderie. It is so much more than the actual prospect of catching a fish. Most of the time we didn't bring a fish home. Well, my brother and I didn't.

Mental: I am the kind of person who must be challenged. I thrive on it. Demand it in my work environment. Expect it in most activities I undertake. I stagnate if not mentally piqued. I'm no Einstein, not even close, but that doesn't negate my need for mental stimulation. It can be as simple as a crossword puzzle, to a complex idea that must be analyzed and thought through. I like to puzzle the unknown and the possible. I find satisfaction when I can sit down with friends and talk about an idea and critique it from all angles, with no holds barred. I'm a huge fan of *In Search Of* and other programs that delve into the unknown. My favorite television channels are: The Discovery Channel, The Learning Channel, Animal Planet, The

History Channel and the Travel Channel. PBS also offers some intriguing programs from time to time. I love to read the books by authors who mix the possible with the unknown and/or the near-possible and weave a story that makes me question concepts and accepted patterns of the world around us.

Emotional: Though I have always been told: *You are a strong person, Kathy.* And in some cases that may be true. I believe much of what others think to be a strong character is really just the outward show of my defense mechanisms. I find this more true in the years when I have not had a significant other to share my life with. When on my own, I tend to erect mental barriers. They serve to protect me. And though they may make me appear to be tough and unbreakable, those barriers are not impenetrable. They often protect aspects of my nature that have in the past been deeply

injured and are not yet ready for
public viewing. But back to the
comment about my being strong. I
have to admit that in the last
year I have surmounted some
obstacles that, at the time, I
felt I was not strong enough to
face. There are times when
strength wells up from previously
unknown sources within myself. And
from sources created for me by the
loving gestures of others.
Anxieties and worries have been
apart of my life from the get-go.
I've been called a worrywart since
elementary school. This aspect of
my nature, my tendency towards
nervousness and anxieties, I have
worked on. It has been a slow
process but I have made progress.
I am pleased with the headway I
have made and continue to make.
But being an emotional person has
its plusses. I love to express
myself, to free my emotions. I
like to laugh, to smile, to be
silly, to feel it is okay to growl
outloud if frustrated, to express
love, to receive love, to make

people laugh and smile, to ease
other people's heartache and
burdens, to encourage others to
feel comfortable in my presence--
comfortable enough to express
themselves emotionally.

Tangible (my definition): The
smile of a loved one. The sound of
a belly-born laugh that rumbles
from your tummy and explodes
through your lips in a blasting
guffaw. The ever precious, genuine
giggle of a child. The smell of
fresh cut grass. The fragrance of
wet concrete and rain brushed
vegetation after the first
rainfall of the season. The warm
and strong embrace of a loved one.
The smell of print on the pages of
a new book. The sounds of family
all gathered together; talking,
laughing, even snoring. The spread
of cool sheets on my bed on hot
summer nights. Warm, snuggy
flannel jammies. Wood smoke and
campfires. The susurration of a
wave as it brushes past pebbles,
over sand then draws back from the

shore to do it again. The tang of pines. And the spicy smell of a zephyr as it skims the surface of the briny ocean then rushes past me like a spirit driven onward. The glow of Christmas lights on a misty winter's eve. Puppy breath. The rumble of a Harley Davidson motorcycle. Coyotes howling at sunset from the hills around the lake. The mournful melody and haunting voice of bagpipes. Fireworks bursting from the canopy of night on the Fourth of July. The beat of drums reverberating in my belly as a marching band passes in front of me in a parade. Windchimes and waterfalls. The remembered smell of Dove soap on the hands of my grandmother. The aroma of frying potatoes and onions. Fresh brewed coffee. The feel of warm, soft fur 'neath my palm when I caress my dog or cat. The bark of welcome when I enter the house. The spinning, meowing welcome home from my cat. The twitching eyelids, small whimpers, and running paws of one of my fur

kin when they are dreaming. The
wet, licky kisses placed on my
hand, just because they love me.
The purr of my cat merely because
I am nearby. Wagging tails and
toothy grins. Grasping paws and
thumping tails.

Chapter 21

LIFE GOES ON

Lock the door, or leave it open.
Life goes on whether you do, or
not. Accept it. If you accept it,
do so with a smile. It can't hurt.

I don't know what the future holds
for me. I don't know if there are
darker moments in store in the
months and years ahead. If I
haven't faced the darkest moments,
I know I will not be alone. I have
read the stories. Heard the
accounts of persons who have
suffered heartbreaking losses.
I've heard the true tales of those
who have suffered through bouts of

cancer, not once or twice, but a handful of times.

I look at the world I live in. Others have lived in it--years ago. In the future, more people will live in it. I know that much of what I see has been there for many, many years--before my time: trees, hills and mountains, lakes and streams, cities and farmland. I probably see pretty much what others saw a century ago. And it is likely much will still remain the same, look the same now as it will a century from now. Rather puts my life into perspective. I still drive and walk down the streets and sidewalks my father traveled on, my grandparents, too. And my father and grandparents are, now, many years gone from this earth. I glance around me at the young people. When I'm gone their eyes will look upon many of the same landscapes I have seen. Places that have become familiar to me. Places I could describe as from the details of a picture.

More exacting--the world goes on, and life in whatever form it exists in goes on, too. Not going to change that. But I can live it, every day, for as long as I am here. The world around me is there for me--today. Now. The past is beyond my grasp. The future, too. I will *only* have today. It is no different for every person on this globe, young or old or middle aged. This is my time and it is no less substantial than any life lived a lifetime ago, or a century ago.

I hope I live it well, honorably, and fully.

THANK YOU...

God, for giving me life, a family to love, friends to cherish, and an imagination that keeps me on my toes.

To the dear doctors who gave me
hope, honesty, healing... new
life.

Greg and Terri Bacchetti for your
support and strength. Thank you
for the laughs and long talks.
Thank you, Greg, for drumming over
and over, for fifteen years, how
special Golden Retrievers are.
Thank you both for your part in
reuniting our group of family and
friends.

Paula and Larry Graves, my
longtime friends. You have
accepted me in all my expressions
of life--all the years, through
many changes. You have seen the
secret places in my heart and
smiled with affection and
understanding.

Daniel Terzian. You have been one
of the best examples of strength
in the human flesh I have ever
known. I have looked to your
example to shape my own growth.
Thank you for sharing your joys of

"fatherhood" of the two felines in your keep. Thank you for your undisguised enjoyment of life. Thank you for opening the night skies to my eyes and mind and in so doing feeding my ever questing imagination.

Randy, my brother, for your unshakable love and support. I have felt your comforting presence even though you are usually many miles away. Thank you for your quiet and gentle love.

Mom, my dearest friend. I don't even know where to begin to offer up all the thanks you deserve. Had it not been for you, I doubt I'd be here now. When I was faced with my darkest moments, you opened the door and brought all the bright light in, banishing my demons and lifting me up with your loving, generous, never flagging spirit. You are the embodiment of the heart, backbone, and soul of a mother.

Ken, the father I wouldn't have
had these past twenty-one years,
had you not asked my mother to
marry you. In you I have found the
friendship a daughter can have
with a father--the kind that is
developed once the child is an
adult. I am proud to call you Dad.
I am glad I have a father to share
my adult years with. Thank you for
filling that space and for being
my friend, too.

My furry companions. You share my
personal world more than any other
living thing. You are there when I
get home from work. Beside me as I
lay down to sleep. Concerned about
me when I am ill, or sad. Happy to
share every moment with me,
regardless of what we are doing.
You ask so little and give so
much. You fill my every day with
your boundless spirits, clownish
personalities, and your good and
pure hearts. It is a pleasure to
wake up to your thumping tails,
purring coos, and ever happy
natures. And when I am away from

home, you warm my heart and keep
me company in my thoughts. Hugs
for you all!

* * *

About the Author:

Kathy lives in California, where
she shares her life with her
husband and furry family. She
finds inspiration for her novels,
short stories, and poems from her
family, her past jobs, her life's
experiences -- from a diagnosis of
cancer, twice -- to a diagnosis of
life, and from the furry loved
ones who share her world. Much of
Kathy's work reflects her
enthusiasm for the magic of music,
the enchantment of the Earth and
the beauty of all creatures
dwelling in our midst. She writes
to reach the reader's heart and
mind and make a difference.

The author has been writing since
her youth; four decades and
counting. She has been a student
of the martial arts; and while

attending university studied anthropology, mythology and folklore. Kathy has six published books. She is also a contributing author for the much anticipated book: Inspiring Generations: 150 Years, 150 Stories in Yosemite - released May 13, 2014. In addition, some of her stories are featured in other various well-known anthologies. Her award-winning poetry and short stories have been featured in online publications and traditional hard-copy print such as newspapers, books and magazines.

Recently retired, Kathy is now able to pursue her full-time writing career.